C000165731

# Keto Recipes for a Delicious Dinner

## A Keto Cookbook for Enjoying a Tasty Dinner with no Regrets

By Carla Wilson

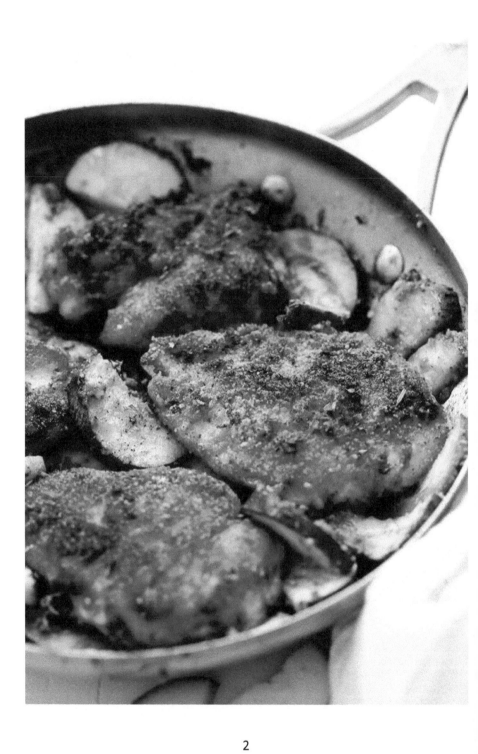

content within this book has been derived from various sources. Please consult a licensed professional before attempting any techniques outlined in this book.

By reading this document, the reader agrees that under no circumstances is the author responsible for any losses, direct or indirect, which are incurred as a result of the use of information contained within this document, including, but not limited to, — errors, omissions, or inaccuracies.

# Table of Contents

7

# Zucchini Lasagna with Meat Sauce

**Preparation Time:** 10 minutes

**Cooking Time:** 6 hours

**Servings:** 6

**Ingredients:**

- 4 small zucchinis, ends cut off (you can sub two large zucchinis)
- 1 pound(500gr) cooked ground meat or chopped meatballs
- 1/2 cup of your favorite pasta sauce
- 8 oz. mozzarella cheese, freshly shredded (about 2 cups), divided
- 15oz (425gr) container of part-skim ricotta cheese
- 1/2 cup Parmesan cheese, freshly grated - 2 eggs
- 1 tablespoon dried parsley flakes
- 1 teaspoon salt
- 1/2 teaspoon cracked black pepper

**Directions:**

1. Thinly slice (unpeeled) zucchini length-wise into thin strips, like lasagna noodles. It's easier to do this with a mandolin, but a large knife works just fine. (It's OK if some are only a few inches long.) Create cheese filling

by combining 1 cup mozzarella cheese, ricotta cheese, Parmesan cheese, eggs, parsley flakes, salt, and pepper.

2. Create a layer of zucchini at the bottom of your slow cooker. (It's OK if pieces overlap.)

3. Top zucchini with a rounded 1/2 cup of cheese filling, 1 cup meat, and 1-3 tablespoons sauce.

4. Continue layering zucchini, cheese, meat, and sauce until you only have enough zucchini left for top layer. (A 6-quart slow cooker will have 4-5 layers and a 4-quart slow cooker will have 6-8 layers.)

5. Before you add the top layer of zucchini, add whatever sauce, meat, and cheese you have left. Top with zucchini and remaining 1 cup of mozzarella cheese.

6. Cover, and cook on low for 6-8 hours. Turn off slow cooker and let rest for at least 30 minutes, so juices become more set.

## Nutrition:

- 386 calories
- 23.4g fat
- 112g protein

# Chinese Pulled Pork – Char Siu

**Preparation Time:** 10 minutes

**Cooking Time:** 7 hours

**Servings:** 6

**Ingredients:**

- 1 kg pork shoulder or loin
- 1 cup chicken broth homemade is best
- 4 tablespoons sugar free tomato sauce homemade is best
- 1 tablespoon tomato paste
- 2 tablespoons garlic paste
- 4 tablespoons soy sauce
- 5 drops liquid sweetener
- 2 teaspoons ginger paste
- 1 teaspoon smoked paprika

**Directions:**

1. Place the pork in the bottom of the slow cooker. Combine all remaining ingredients and pour over the pork, ensuring it gets underneath as well.
2. Cook on low for 7 hours. Shred the pork with a fork and stir through the sauce, cooking for a further 30 - 60 minutes until the sauce has thickened to your liking, or eat it straight away.

## Nutrition:

- 392 calories
- 23g fat
- 31g protein

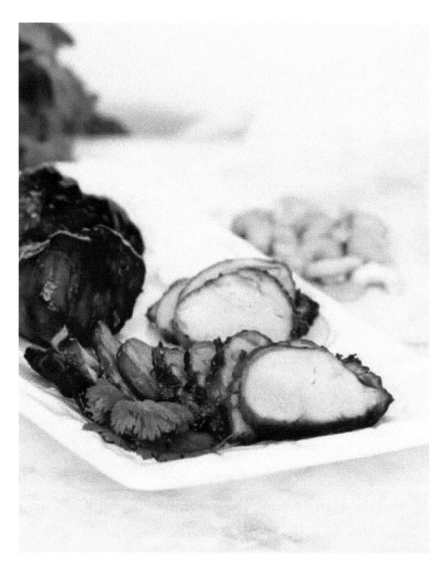

# Garlic Butter Chicken with Cream Cheese Sauce

**Preparation Time:** 10 minutes

**Cooking Time:** 7 hours

**Servings:** 6

**Ingredients:**

*For the garlic chicken:*

- 2- 2.5 lbs. of chicken breasts
- 1 stick of butter
- 8 garlic cloves, sliced in half to release flavor
- 1 tsp. salt
- Optional (but recommended) – 1 sliced onion or 2 tsps. of onion powder

*For the cream cheese sauce:*

- 8 oz. of cream cheese
- 1 cup of chicken stock
- salt to taste

**Directions:**

1. for the garlic chicken:
2. Place the chicken (thawed) in the slow cooker. Add the butter to the slow cooker. Place the garlic in the slow cooker, dispersing it around so it's not all in one spot.

13

Sprinkle with salt. Cook on low for 6 hours. Remove and place on serving platter

3. for the cream cheese sauce:

4. In a pan, put the cup of chicken stock (or liquid from the slow cooker). Add the cream cheese and salt. Cook over medium-low heat until the sauce is combined and creamy. Pour over chicken.

**Nutrition:**

- 664 calories
- 38g fat
- 63g protein

# Spinach Artichoke Chicken

**Preparation Time:** 10 minutes

**Cooking Time:** 4 hours

**Servings:** 6

**Ingredients:**

- 16 oz. Cream Cheese softened
- 9 oz. Frozen Spinach cooked and drained well
- 14.5 oz. Artichoke Hearts chopped
- 1 tbsp. garlic
- 2 cups shredded mozzarella
- 3 lbs. boneless, skinless chicken (we used thighs)
- salt and pepper to taste

**Directions:**

1. Place the chicken in the bottom of a slow cooker. Salt and Pepper well. In a bowl, mix together cream cheese, spinach, artichokes, garlic and season with salt and pepper.
2. Stir in mozzarella cheese. Cook on low for 4-5 hours.

**Nutrition:**

- 460 calories
- 10g fat
- 34g protein

# Bacon Wrapped Pork Loin

**Preparation Time:** 10 minutes

**Cooking Time:** 7 hours

**Servings:** 4

**Ingredients:**

- 2 lb. pork loin roast
- 4 strips uncooked bacon
- 1 package dry onion soup mix
- 1/4 cup water

**Directions:**

1. Rub pork loin with the dry onion soup mix. Pour any leftover into the bottom of the crock pot (any that fell off on my cutting board I scraped into mine).
2. Wrap the bacon around the roast and place into the crock pot. Pour in the water. Cook on High for 5 hours or Low for 7.

**Nutrition:**

- 388 calories
- 19g fat
- 40g protein

# Chicken Cordon Bleu with Cauliflower

**Preparation Time:** 10 minutes

**Cooking Time:** 45 minutes

**Servings:** 4

**Ingredients:**

- 4 boneless chicken breast halves (about 12 ounces)
- 4 slices deli ham
- 4 slices Swiss cheese
- 1 large egg, whisked well
- 2 ounces pork rinds
- ¼ cup almond flour
- ¼ cup grated parmesan cheese
- ½ teaspoon garlic powder
- Salt and pepper
- 2 cups cauliflower florets

**Directions:**

1. Preheat the oven to 350 ° F and add a foil on a baking sheet. Sandwich the breast half of the chicken between parchment parts and pound flat. Spread the bits out and cover with ham and cheese sliced over.
2. Roll the chicken over the fillings and then dip into the beaten egg. In a food processor, mix the pork rinds,

almond flour, parmesan, garlic powder, salt and pepper, and pulse into fine crumbs.

3. Roll the rolls of chicken in the mixture of pork rind then put them on the baking sheet. Throw the cauliflower into the baking sheet with the melted butter and fold. Bake for 45 minutes until the chicken is fully cooked.

**Nutrition:**

- 420 Calories
- 23g Fats
- 7g Protein

# Sesame-Crusted Tuna with Green Beans

**Preparation Time:** 15 minutes

**Cooking Time:** 5 minutes

**Servings:** 4

**Ingredients:**

- ¼ cup white sesame seeds
- ¼ cup black sesame seeds
- 4 (6-ounce) Ahi tuna steaks
- Salt and pepper
- 1 tablespoon olive oil
- 1 tablespoon coconut oil
- 2 cups green beans

**Directions:**

1. In a shallow dish, mix the two kinds of sesame seeds. Season the tuna with pepper and salt. Dredge the tuna in a mixture of sesame seeds. Heat up to high heat the olive oil in a skillet, then add the tuna.

2. Cook for 1 to 2 minutes until it turns seared, then sear on the other side. Remove the tuna from the skillet, and let the tuna rest while using the coconut oil to heat the skillet. Fry the green beans in the oil for 5 minutes then use sliced tuna to eat.

# Nutrition:

- 370 Calories
- 23g Fats
- 7g Protein

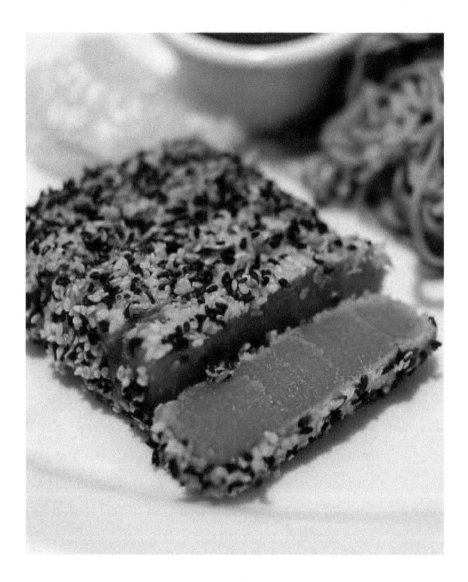

# Rosemary Roasted Pork with Cauliflower

**Preparation Time:** 10 minutes

**Cooking Time:** 20 minutes

**Servings:** 4

**Ingredients:**

- 1 ½ pounds boneless pork tenderloin
- 1 tablespoon coconut oil
- 1 tablespoon fresh chopped rosemary
- Salt and pepper
- 1 tablespoon olive oil
- 2 cups cauliflower florets

**Directions:**

1. Rub the coconut oil into the pork, then season with the rosemary, salt, and pepper. Heat up the olive oil over medium to high heat in a large skillet.
2. Add the pork on each side and cook until browned for 2 to 3 minutes. Sprinkle the cauliflower over the pork in the skillet.
3. Reduce heat to low, then cover the skillet and cook until the pork is cooked through for 8 to 10 minutes. Slice the pork with cauliflower and eat.

**Nutrition:**

- 320 Calories
- 37g Fats
- 3g Protein:

# Grilled Salmon and Zucchini with Mango Sauce

**Preparation Time:** 5 minutes

**Cooking Time:** 10 minutes

**Servings:** 4

**Ingredients:**

- 4 (6-ounce) boneless salmon fillets
- 1 tablespoon olive oil
- Salt and pepper
- 1 large zucchini, sliced in coins
- 2 tablespoons fresh lemon juice
- ½ cup chopped mango
- ¼ cup fresh chopped cilantro
- 1 teaspoon lemon zest
- ½ cup canned coconut milk

**Directions:**

1. Preheat a grill pan to heat, and sprinkle with cooking spray liberally. Brush with olive oil to the salmon and season with salt and pepper.
2. Apply lemon juice to the zucchini, and season with salt and  pepper. Put the zucchini and salmon fillets on the grill pan.

3. Cook for 5 minutes then turn all over and cook for another 5 minutes.
4. Combine the remaining ingredients in a blender and combine to create a sauce. Serve the side-drizzled salmon filets with mango sauce and zucchini.

**Nutrition:**

- 350 Calories
- 23g Fats
- 7g Protein
- 6g Carbohydrates

# Beef and Broccoli Stir-Fry

**Preparation Time:** 20 minutes

**Cooking Time:** 15 minutes

**Servings:** 4

**Ingredients:**

- ¼ cup soy sauce
- 1 tablespoon sesame oil
- 1 teaspoon garlic chili paste
- 1-pound beef sirloin
- 2 tablespoons almond flour
- 2 tablespoons coconut oil
- 2 cups chopped broccoli florets
- 1 tablespoon grated ginger
- 3 cloves garlic, minced

**Directions:**

1. In a small bowl, whisk the soy sauce, sesame oil, and chili paste together. In a plastic freezer bag, slice the beef and mix with the almond flour. Pour in the sauce and toss to coat for 20 minutes, then let rest.

2. Heat up the oil over medium to high heat in a large skillet. In the pan, add the beef and sauce and cook until the beef is browned.

3. Move the beef to the skillet sides, then add the broccoli, ginger, and garlic. Sauté until tender-crisp broccoli, then throw it all together and serve hot.

**Nutrition:**

- 350 Calories 19g Fats
- 37g Protein
- 6g Carbohydrates

# Parmesan-Crusted Halibut with Asparagus

**Preparation Time:** 10 minutes

**Cooking Time:** 15 minutes

**Servings:** 4

**Ingredients:**

- 2 tablespoons olive oil
- ¼ cup butter, softened
- Salt and pepper
- ¼ cup grated Parmesan
- 1-pound asparagus, trimmed
- 2 tablespoons almond flour
- 4 (6-ounce) boneless halibut fillets
- 1 teaspoon garlic powder

**Directions:**

1. Preheat the oven to 400 F and line a foil-based baking sheet. Throw the asparagus in olive oil and scatter over the baking sheet.

2. In a blender, add the butter, Parmesan cheese, almond flour, garlic powder, salt and pepper, and mix until smooth. Place the fillets with the asparagus on the baking sheet, and spoon the Parmesan over the eggs.

3. Bake for 10 to 12 minutes, then broil until browned for 2 to 3 minutes.

## Nutrition:

- 415 Calories
- 26g Fats
- 42g Protein
- 3g Carbohydrates

# Hearty Beef and Bacon Casserole

**Preparation Time:** 25 minutes

**Cooking Time:** 30 minutes

**Servings:** 8

**Ingredients:**

- 8 slices uncooked bacon
- 1 medium head cauliflower, chopped
- ¼ cup canned coconut milk
- Salt and pepper
- 2 pounds ground beef (80% lean)
- 8 ounces mushrooms, sliced
- 1 large yellow onion, chopped
- 2 cloves garlic, minced

**Directions:**

1. Preheat to 375 F on the oven. Cook the bacon in a skillet until crispy, then drain and chop on paper towels.
2. Bring to boil a pot of salted water, then add the cauliflower. Boil until tender for 6 to 8 minutes then drain and add the coconut milk to a food processor. Mix until smooth, then sprinkle with salt and pepper.
3. Cook the beef until browned in a pan, then wash the fat away. Remove the mushrooms, onion, and garlic,

then move to a baking platter. Place on top of the cauliflower mixture and bake for 30 minutes. Broil for 5 minutes on high heat, then sprinkle with bacon to serve.

## Nutrition:

- 410 Calories
- 25g Fats
- 37g Protein
- 6g Carbohydrates

# Sesame Wings with Cauliflower

**Preparation Time:** 5 minutes

**Cooking Time:** 30 minutes

**Servings:** 4

**Ingredients:**

- 2 ½ tablespoons soy sauce
- 2 tablespoons sesame oil
- 1 ½ teaspoons balsamic vinegar
- 1 teaspoon minced garlic
- 1 teaspoon grated ginger
- Salt
- 1-pound chicken wing, the wings itself
- 2 cups cauliflower florets

**Directions:**

1. In a freezer bag, mix the soy sauce, sesame oil, balsamic vinegar, garlic, ginger, and salt, then add the chicken wings. Coat flip, then chill for 2 to 3 hours.
2. Preheat the oven to 400 F and line a foil-based baking sheet. Spread the wings along with the cauliflower onto the baking sheet. Bake for 35 minutes, then sprinkle on to serve with sesame seeds.

# Nutrition:

- 400 Calories
- 15g Fats
- 5g Protein
- 3g Carbohydrates

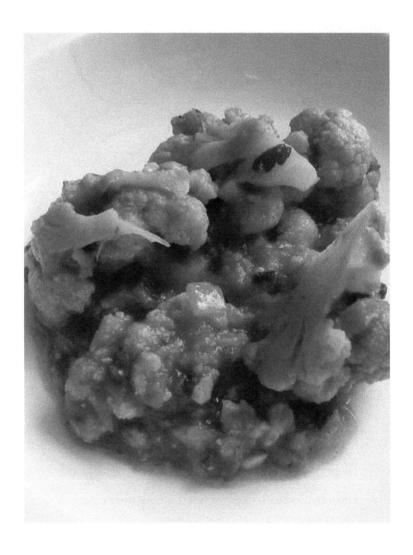

# Fried Coconut Shrimp with Asparagus

**Preparation Time:** 15 minutes

**Cooking Time:** 10 minutes

**Servings:** 6

**Ingredients:**

- 1 ½ cups shredded unsweetened coconut - 2 large eggs
- Salt and pepper
- 1 ½ pounds large shrimp, peeled and deveined
- ½ cup canned coconut milk
- 1-pound asparagus, cut into 2-inch pieces

**Directions:**

1. Pour the coconut onto a shallow platter. Beat the eggs in a bowl with a little salt and pepper. Dip the shrimp into the egg first, then dredge with coconut.

2. Heat up coconut oil over medium-high heat in a large skillet. Add the shrimp and fry over each side for 1 to 2 minutes until browned.

3. Remove the paper towels from the shrimp and heat the skillet again. Remove the asparagus and sauté to tender-crisp with salt and pepper, then serve with the shrimp.

## Nutrition:

- 535 Calories
- 38g Fats
- 16g Protein
- 3g Carbohydrates

# Coconut Chicken Curry with Cauliflower Rice

**Preparation time:** 15 minutes

**Cooking time:** 30 minutes

**Servings:** 6

**Ingredients:**

- 1 tablespoon olive oil
- 1 medium yellow onion, chopped
- 1 ½ pounds boneless chicken thighs, chopped
- Salt and pepper
- 1 (14-ounce) can coconut milk
- 1 tablespoon curry powder
- 1 ¼ teaspoon ground turmeric
- 3 cups riced cauliflower

**Directions:**

1. Heat the oil over medium heat, in a large skillet. Add the onions, and cook for about 5 minutes, until translucent.

2. Stir in the chicken and season with salt and pepper-cook for 6 to 8 minutes, stirring frequently until all sides are browned. Pour the coconut milk into the pan, then whisk in the curry and turmeric powder.

3. Simmer until hot and bubbling, for 15 to 20 minutes. Meanwhile, steam the cauliflower rice until tender with a few tablespoons of water. Serve the cauliflower rice over the curry.

**Nutrition:**

- 430 Calories
- 29g Fats
- 9g Protein
- 3g Carbohydrates

# Grilled Whole Chicken

**Preparation Time:** 20 minutes

**Cooking Time:** 20 minutes

**Servings:** 6

**Ingredients:**

- ¼ cup butter
- 2 tablespoons lemon juice
- 2 teaspoons fresh lemon zest
- 1 teaspoon dried oregano
- 2 teaspoons paprika
- 1 teaspoon onion powder
- 1 teaspoon garlic powder
- Salt and ground black pepper
- 1 (4-pound) grass-fed whole chicken

**Directions:**

1. Preheat the grill to medium heat. Grease the grill grate. Place onto a large cutting board, breast-side down. Mix butter, lemon juice, lemon zest, oregano, spices, salt, and black pepper.
2. Cut both sides of backbone. Remove the backbone. Flip and open. Firmly press breast to flatten.
3. Coat the whole chicken with the oil mixture. Grill for 20 minutes.

4. Remove from the grill and set aside for 10 minutes.

**Nutrition:**

- 532 Calories
- 17g Fat
- 0.5g Fiber

# Grilled Chicken Breast

**Preparation Time:** 15 minutes

**Cooking Time:** 14 minutes

**Servings:** 4

**Ingredients:**

- ¼ cup balsamic vinegar
- 2 tablespoons olive oil
- 1½ teaspoons lemon juice
- ½ teaspoon lemon-pepper seasoning
- 4 (6-ounce) grass-fed chicken breast halves

**Directions:**

1. Blend vinegar, oil, lemon juice, and seasoning. Coat chicken breasts with the mixture. Marinate for 30 minutes.
2. Preheat and grease the grill to medium heat. Place the chicken breasts onto the grill and cover.
3. Cook for 7 minutes. Serve.

**Nutrition:**

- 258 Calories
- 11.3g Fat
- 0.1g Fiber

# Glazed Chicken Thighs

**Preparation Time:** 15 minutes

**Cooking Time:** 35 minutes

**Servings:** 8

**Ingredients:**

- ½ cup balsamic vinegar
- 1/3 cup low-sodium soy sauce
- 3 tablespoons Yukon syrup
- 4 tablespoons olive oil
- 3 tablespoons chili sauce
- 2 tablespoons garlic
- Salt and black pepper
- 8 (6-ounce) grass-fed chicken thighs

**Directions:**

1. Mix all ingredients (except chicken thighs and sesame seeds). Mix half of marinade and chicken thighs. Seal and shake well.
2. Chill for 1 hour. Chill remaining marinade. Preheat oven to 425°F.
3. Mix reserved marinade over medium heat and boil. Cook for 5 minutes. Remove and set aside.

4. Remove from the bag and discard excess marinade. Arrange chicken thighs into a 9x13-inch baking dish in a single layer and coat with cooked marinade.

5. Bake for 30 minutes. Serve.

**Nutrition:**

- 406 Calories
- 19.6g Fat
- 0.1g Fiber

# Bacon-Wrapped Chicken Breasts

**Preparation Time:** 15 minutes

**Cooking Time:** 33 minutes Servings: 4

**Ingredients :**

**Chicken Marinade:**

- 3 tablespoons balsamic vinegar
- 3 tablespoons olive oil
- 2 tablespoons water
- 1 garlic clove
- 1 teaspoon dried Italian seasoning
- ½ teaspoon dried rosemary
- 4 (6-ounce) grass-fed chicken breasts

**Stuffing:**

- 16 fresh basil leaves
- 1 large fresh tomato
- 4 provolone cheese slices
- 8 bacon slices
- ¼ cup Parmesan cheese

**Directions:**

1. For marinade:
   a. Mix all ingredients (except chicken).
2. For chicken

3. Chop chicken breast horizontally, without cutting all the way through.
4. Repeat with the remaining chicken breasts. Coat with marinade. Chill 30 minutes.
5. Preheat your oven to 500°F. Grease baking dish.
6. Place 4 basil leaves onto the bottom half of a chicken breast. Followed by 3 tomato slices and 1 provolone cheese slice. Fold the top half over filling.
7. Wrap the breast with 3 bacon slices. Repeat. Situate into the prepared baking dish in a single layer.
8. Bake for 30 minutes. Remove and sprinkle with Parmesan cheese evenly. Bake for 3 minutes more.

**Nutrition:**

- 633 Calories
- 36g Fat
- 0.3g Fiber

# Chicken Parmigiana

**Preparation Time:** 15 minutes

**Cooking Time:** 26 minutes

**Servings:** 5

**Ingredients:**

- 5 (6-ounce) grass-fed chicken breasts
- 1 large organic egg
- ½ cup superfine almond flour
- ¼ cup Parmesan cheese,
- ½ teaspoon dried parsley
- ½ teaspoon paprika
- ½ teaspoon garlic powder
- 1 cup sugar-free tomato sauce
- 5 ounces mozzarella cheese
- 2 tablespoons fresh parsley

**Directions:**

1. Preheat your oven to 375°F. Wrap 1 chicken breast in parchment paper. Pound the chicken breast into ½-inch thickness
2. Repeat with the rest. Put the beaten egg. Mix almond flour, Parmesan, parsley, spices, salt, and black pepper in another dish.

3. Dip it into the whipped egg and coat with the flour mixture. Heat the oil over medium-high heat and fry for 3 minutes.

4. Dry chicken breasts. Spread at bottom of a casserole dish ½ cup of tomato sauce. Arrange the chicken breasts over marinara sauce in a single layer.

5. Drizzle with the remaining tomato sauce, mozzarella cheese slices. Bake for 20 minutes. Garnish with parsley. Serve

**Nutrition:**

- 458 Calories
- 25.4g Fat
- 7.9g Carbs

# Beef and Eggplant Kebab

**Preparation Time:** 20 minutes

**Cooking Time:** 15 minutes

**Serving:** 4

**Ingredients:**

- 3 tbsp. oil
- 1/2 tsp. dried thyme
- 1/2 tsp. oregano
- 2 eggs (beaten)
- 1/2 eggplant
- 1/2 tsp. chili pepper (ground)
- 1/4 cup olive oil
- 4 garlic cloves (crushed)
- 1 cup parsley leaves (chopped)
- 1 lb. beef (minced)
- 1 tsp. salt
- 1/2 tsp. black pepper

**Directions:**

1. Cut the eggplant into thin slices of about half inch. Season with salt and set aside. Put minced meat in a large bowl, add thyme, eggs, chili pepper, onions,

parsley, olive oil, garlic, salt, oregano, and black pepper.

2. Combine the mixture. Shape equal-sized patties with wet hands. Preheat a skillet over medium-high heat and grease with oil. Rinse the eggplant slices sprinkled with salt and pat dry with hand or paper towel. Thread eggplant slices and patties alternately onto skewers and place on the preheated skillet.

3. Flip the sides occasionally and cook for 15 minutes. Remove from the heat and garnish with parsley. Serve warm with low-carb pita bread.

## Nutrition:

- 39g Fat
- 23g Protein
- 4g Net Carbs
- 465 Calories

# Skin Salmon with Pesto Cauliflower Rice

**Preparation Time:** 20 minutes

**Cooking Time:** 20 minutes

**Serving:** 3

**Ingredients:**

- 3 cups frozen riced cauliflower
- 1/cup olive oil
- 1 lemon
- 1 scoop keto MCT powder
- 1/4 cup hemp hearts
- 3 garlic cloves
- 3 salmon fillets
- 1 tbsp. butter
- 1 tbsp. olive oil
- 1 tbsp. coconut amino
- 1 tsp. red boat fish sauce
- 1 cup basil leaves (chopped)
- 1/2 tsp. pink salt
- Pinch of salt

**Directions:**

1. Grease a dish with olive oil, add coconut amino and fish sauce. Pat dry the salmon fillets and place them on

marinade with meat side down. Season the top with salt and set aside for about 20 minutes. Add the minced garlic, hemp hearts, lemon juice, basil, olive oil, MCT powder, and salt in a food processor.

2. Blend until it reaches a sauce-like consistency. Add olive oil to a large skillet and put it on the stove-top. Add the cauliflower rice and cook until crisp-tender. Scoop out a few spoons of pesto you prepared and add into the skillet. Season with pink salt and stir until fully incorporated.

3. Place a skillet on medium heat and line with butter. Add the salmon with skin side down and cook for 5 minutes or until the crust browns. Flip the side and coat it with the remaining marinade. Sauté for about 2 minutes and remove from heat. Dish out the salmon and cauliflower rice. Top with pesto and serve warm.

**Nutrition:**

- 51 g Fat
- 33.8g Protein
- 10g Net Carbs
- 647 Calories

# Chicken Enchilada Casserole

**Preparation Time:** 5 minutes

**Cooking Time:** 40 minutes

**Serving:** 6

**Ingredients:**

- 1/4 tsp. xanthan gum
- 1/2 tsp. onion powder
- 1 tsp. chili powder
- 1 tsp. cumin
- 1 tsp. garlic powder
- 1 tsp. oregano
- 6 lbs. chicken breast (boneless)
- 2 oz. black olives (slivered)
- 2 cups chicken broth
- 4 oz. green chilies
- 3/4 cup sour cream
- 1 cup cheddar cheese
- 3 tbsp. butter
- 1/2 tsp. pink Himalayan salt

**Directions:**

1. Place a large skillet over medium-high heat and add butter. Add the xanthan gum and allow thickening.

Pour the chicken broth and stir through the xanthan gum. Allow cooking for two minutes. Sprinkle with salt, onion powder, olive, cumin, and oregano, and chilies. Stir thoroughly to combine.

2. Add the chicken and bring to boil. Low the flame and allow cooking for 20 minutes with the lid on. Stir occasionally to avoid sticking. Remove from heat once the chicken is fully cooked. Shred the cooked chicken into small chunks. Place a skillet over medium heat and add in the sour cream. Stir in the spices to taste and add the shredded chicken. Preheat the oven to 350°F. Season with cheddar cheese and transfer the skillet to the oven. Bake for 10 minutes or until the cheese melts. Serve warm with cauliflower rice or tortillas.

3. Keep in an airtight container to refrigerate for up to two weeks.

**Nutrition:**

- 20.7g Fat
- 27.8g Protein
- 4.5g Net Carbs
- 309 Calories

# Keto Cottage Pie

**Preparation Time:** 15 minutes

**Cooking Time:** 45 minutes

**Serving:** 10

**Ingredients:**

*Base:*

- 2 pounds beef (minced)
- 3 celery sticks (chopped)
- 1 onion (chopped)
- 1 tbsp. dried oregano
- 2 garlic cloves (ground)
- 3 tbsp. olive oil
- 3 tbsp. tomato paste
- 1 cup beef stock
- 1/4 cup red wine vinegar
- 2 tbsp. dried thyme leaves
- 10 ounces green beans
- 1 tsp. salt

*Topping:*

- 3 ounces butter
- 1 pinch of dried oregano
- 3 eggs (only yolk)

- 1/4 tsp. pepper (ground)
- 6 pounds florets of cauliflower
- 1 pinch of paprika
- 1/2 tsp. salt

## Directions:

1. Put a large skillet over medium-high flame. Add olive oil, oregano, onion, celery, and garlic. Grill for 5 minutes or until the onion becomes translucent.

2. Add the minced beef and sprinkle salt. Stir occasionally till the meat begins to brown. Add tomato paste to the cooked meat and mix well. Pour the beef stock and red wine vinegar.

3. Allow stewing for 20 minutes till the stock and vinegar evaporate. Add thyme and green beans and cook for another 5 minutes. Use a slotted spoon to dish out the mixture and set aside.

4. Take a large saucepan and fill two-third of it with water. Cover the pan and heat till the water begins to boil. Add the cauliflower florets to boiling water. Simmer for about 7 minutes until it tenders.

5. Discard the cooking water carefully.

6. Add butter, pepper, and salt to the saucepan containing drained cauliflower.

7. Mash the tendered cauliflower by stick blender. Add egg yolks to the mashed cauliflower and mix well.

8. Preheat the oven to 350°F. Grease the baking dish with butter and transfer the minced beef mixture to it.

9. Top it with cauliflower mash. Garnish with oregano and paprika. Bake in preheated oven for half an hour or until the top starts to brown. Serve immediately or refrigerate for up to 7 days.

**Nutrition:**

- 36g Fat
- 18g Protein
- 4g Net Carbs
- 420 Calories

# Pan Fried Spinach Stuffed Chicken

**Preparation Time:** 10 minutes

**Cooking Time:** 20 minutes

**Serving:** 2

**Ingredients:**

- 1 tbsp. mozzarella cheese (grated)
- 2 tbsp. cream cheese
- 1 chicken breast (boneless)
- 1 tbsp. onion (chopped)
- Oil as needed
- 1 tbsp. butter
- 1/2 cup spinach (chopped)
- Salt to taste
- Pepper to taste

**Directions:**

1. Place a pan over medium-high heat and add butter. Add onions and spinach, allow to cook for two minutes or until cooked thoroughly. Add in the cream cheese to the pan, mix well to combine. Allow simmering for two minutes.

2. Lay the chicken flat on your cutting board. Use a sharp knife to deep cut a pocket through chicken breast. Flavor both sides of chicken with salt and pepper.

Spoon the shredded cheese and spinach mixture into the pocket.

3. Fold and seal the chicken breast with toothpicks. Place a skillet over medium-high heat and add olive oil. Cover the pan with a lid and cook the chicken for 8 minutes or until golden. Cut through the middle and serve hot.

**Nutrition:**

- 15g Fat
- 27g Protein
- 255Calories

# Keto Chicken Tenders

**Preparation Time:** 10 minutes

**Cooking Time:** 30 minutes

**Serving:** 6

**Ingredients:**

- 1 egg
- 1 lb. chicken breast tenders
- 1 tbsp. heavy whipping cream
- 6 oz. buffalo sauce
- 1 cup almond flour
- Salt to taste
- Pepper to taste

**Directions:**

1. Preheat the oven to 350°F. Marinate the chicken tenders with salt and pepper. Crack the egg into a small bowl and beat it with heavy cream. Mix the almond flour with salt and pepper in a zip-top bag or mixing bowl.

2. Dip the marinated tender in the egg and then in the almond flour. Repeat the process with all tenders. You can also coat the tenders by shaking them in a Ziploc bag filled with almond flour. Ensure the tenders are well coated with almond flour.

3. Use the fork to place tenders on a baking sheet greased with oil. Place the sheet in the oven and allow to bake for 30 minutes or until the crust browns. Remove from the oven and allow to cool. Add buffalo sauce and tenders in a Tupperware container and shake gently for proper coating. Transfer to the serving plate and enjoy the delicious chicken tenders.

## Nutrition:

- 14.7g Fat
- 29.3g Protein
- 285 Calories

# Low-Carb Salmon Tray Bake

**Preparation Time:** 5 minutes

**Cooking Time:** 15 minutes

**Serving:** 2

**Ingredients:**

- 2 medium salmon fillets
- 1 bunch broccolini
- 1 tbsp. extra virgin olive oil
- 2 tsp. whole-grain mustard
- 4 tbsp. Paleo mayonnaise
- 2 tsp. Dijon mustard
- Salt, to taste
- Black pepper, to taste
- Lemon wedges, to serve

**Directions:**

1. Preheat the oven to 200°C. Lay the broccolini on a cutting board and trim off the inedible parts — place in a baking tray and drizzle with olive oil. Pat the salmon fillets, and sprinkle the top with Dijon and whole-grain mustard.

2. Lay the salmon and lemon wedges with broccolini in the tray — season with salt and pepper. Bake for about 10 minutes until salmon is evenly-cooked, and

broccolini turns tender-crisp. Serve instantly with mayonnaise or store in the refrigerator for one day.

**Nutrition:**

- 42.5g Fat
- 34.3g Protein
- 552 Calories

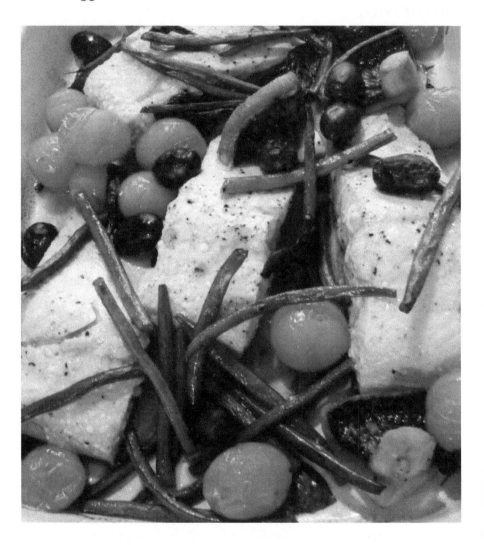

# Zesty Low-Carb Chicken Tacos

**Preparation Time:** 15 minutes

**Cooking Time:** 35 minutes

**Serving:** 4

**Ingredients:**

**Tortillas:**

- 3/4 cup egg whites
- 1/3 cup water
- 1/3 cup water
- 1/4 cup coconut flour
- 1/4 cup almond flour
- 2 tbsp. avocado oil
- 1/2 tsp. salt

**Filling:**

- 1 lime
- 2 cups lettuce
- 1 avocado
- 1 lb. chicken breast

**Directions:**

1. Preheat the oven to 400°F and line a baking dish with parchment paper. Place the chicken on a baking dish and bake for 30 minutes or until fork-tender. Add

water, coconut flour, egg whites, almond flour, salt and oil in a mixing bowl. Whisk together to combine.

2. Leave the batter to rest for 10 minutes till all the ingredients absorb well. Place a skillet over medium-high heat and grease with avocado oil. Take 1/4 cup of batter and add to the skillet. Spread the mixture with a wooden spoon.

3. Cook each side for about 4 minutes, flipping the sides occasionally. Remove from the heat once cooked thoroughly. Prepare all four tortillas by the same process. Place each tortilla on a separate parchment sheet and allow cooling. Slice the lettuce, avocado, and lime. Add the lettuce and avocado to the chicken and season with lime. Stuff the tortillas with chicken and lettuce filling.

**Nutrition:**

- 22g Fat
- 30g Protein
- 348 Calories

# Keto Chicken Doner Kebabs

**Preparation Time:** 20 minutes

**Cooking Time:** 50 minutes

**Serving:** 4

**Ingredients:**

- 4 low carb tortillas
- 1-pound chicken thighs
- 1 tsp. paprika powder
- 1 tsp. cumin powder
- 1 tsp. ground coriander
- 1 tbsp. olive oil
- 1 tbsp. lemon juice
- 2 garlic cloves (minced)
- 2 tbsp. hot sauce
- 4 shreds of cheddar cheese
- 4 tbsp. keto garlic sauce
- 1 cup shredded lettuce
- 2 serves keto Lebanese salad (tabbouleh)
- 1/2 tsp. ground pepper
- 1/2 tsp. onion powder
- 1 tsp. salt

**Directions:**

1. Take a large bowl and add chicken, lemon juice, garlic, oil, and all the spices. Marinate the chicken by keeping it in the fridge  for 3 hours. Refrigerate overnight for better results. Preheat the oven to 390°F.

2. Brush the metal skewers with oil and assemble the marinated chicken on them. Place the prepared skewers on the grill rack lined with foil. Make sure the chicken is not touching the bottom. Flip the skewers periodically and bake for an hour or 50 minutes. Make sure the meat is cooked through.

3. Put the chicken aside and prepare kebabs. Take a tortilla wrap and fill it with tabbouleh, cheddar cheese, garlic sauce, and lettuce. Fill all four wraps equally with the same ingredients. Sliver the chicken and add to the wraps. Embellish with hot sauce and gently roll the wraps.

**Nutrition:**

- 38g Fat
- 33g Protein
- 538 Calories

# Low-Carb Pressure Pot Frittata

**Preparation Time:** 10 minutes

**Cooking Time:** 30 minutes Serving: 8

**Ingredients:**

**Frittata:**

- 8 eggs
- 1/2 cup spinach (chopped)
- 1/4 cup red onion (chopped)
- 1/4 cup bell pepper (diced)
- 1/3 cup heavy whipping cream
- 1/2 cup cheddar cheese (shredded)
- Pinch of black pepper
- 1 tsp. chili powder
- 1 tsp. sea salt

**Topping:**

- 1/4 cup red onion (chopped)
- 1 avocado
- 1 tomato (diced)
- 2 tbsp. spring onion (slivered)
- 1 pickled jalapeno pepper (crushed)
- 1/2 cup sour cream

**Directions:**

1. Take a large bowl and beat together the eggs and heavy cream. Add the black pepper, chili powder, salt, spinach, onion, bell pepper, and cheddar cheese. Give a good mix until all the ingredients blend.

2. Grease a 7-inch baking dish with olive oil and transfer the mixture into it.

3. Fill the bottom of the Pressure Pot with 1 cup of water. Place a trivet over the pot to keep the baking dish above water. Secure the lid, and use the manual button to cook for 12 minutes on high pressure.

4. Leave for 15 minutes till the pressure releases naturally. Remove the lid, once the floating valve drops. Add in the chopped tomatoes, salt and red onion. Mix well. Top the frittata with avocado, sour cream, jalapenos, and spring onion. Slice and serve warm. Refrigerate the leftovers in an airtight container for up to 5 days.

**Nutrition:**

- 17.6g Fat
- 9.4g Protein
- 218 Calories

# Balsamic Chicken Thighs

**Preparation Time:** 15 minutes

**Cooking Time:** 4 hours

**Servings:** 8

**Ingredients:**

- 1 teaspoon garlic powder
- 1 teaspoon dried basil
- 1/2 teaspoon salt
- 1/2 teaspoon pepper
- 2 teaspoons dehydrated onion
- 4 garlic cloves minced
- 1 tablespoon extra-virgin olive oil
- 1/2 cup balsamic vinegar divided
- 8 chicken thighs boneless, skinless
- sprinkle of fresh chopped parsley

**Directions:**

1. Combine the first five dry spices in a small bowl and spread over chicken on both sides. Set aside.
2. Pour olive oil and garlic on the bottom of the slow-cooker. Pour in 1/4 cup balsamic vinegar. Place chicken on top.
3. Sprinkle remaining balsamic vinegar over the chicken. Cover and cook on high for 3 hours if you have a fairly

new slow cooker. If you have an older slow cooker you may need to cook another hour. Sprinkle with fresh parsley on top to serve.

**Nutrition:**

- 285 calories
- 20g fat
- 2g fiber
- 18g protein

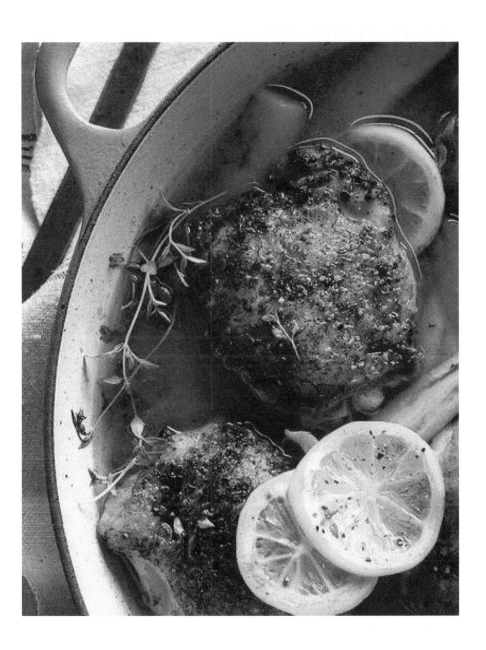

# Chicken Marsala

**Preparation Time:** 15 minutes

**Cooking Time:** 5 hours and 20 minutes

**Servings:** 6

**Ingredients:**

- Cooking spray
- 1 1/2 lb. boneless skinless chicken breasts
- kosher salt
- Freshly ground black pepper
- 8 oz. Mushrooms, sliced
- 3 cloves garlic, minced
- 1 c. marsala wine (you can sub with low-sodium chicken broth in a pinch)
- 1/2 c. water
- 1/4 c. almond flour
- 2 tbsp. heavy cream, optional (to make the sauce creamier)
- 2 tbsp. chopped parsley
- Lemon wedges, for serving

**Directions:**

1. Spray inside of slow-cooker with cooking spray. Season chicken all over with salt and pepper and add

to slow-cooker. Top with mushrooms and garlic then pour Marsala wine on top.

2. Cover and cook on low for 4 to 5 hours, until chicken is cooked through.

3. Remove cooked chicken breasts from slow-cooker. In a small bowl, whisk together water and almond flour and whisk into the sauce. Whisk in heavy cream, if using, then return chicken to slow-cooker. Cover and cook on high until the sauce have thickened, about 20 minutes more. Garnish with parsley and serve with lemon wedges.

**Nutrition:**

- 312 calories
- 5g fat
- 3g fiber
- 33 protein

# Chicken Fajitas

**Preparation Time:** 10 minutes

**Cooking Time:** 3 hours

**Servings:** 6

**Ingredients:**

- 4 boneless, skinless chicken breasts
- 3 bell peppers, thinly sliced
- 1 onion, thinly sliced
- 1/2 (7-oz.) can diced tomatoes
- 2 tsp. cumin
- 1/2 tsp. red pepper flakes
- Kosher salt
- Freshly ground black pepper

**Directions:**

1. Place chicken, bell peppers, and onions in slow-cooker then pour over diced tomatoes. Season with cumin, red pepper flakes, salt, and pepper. Cook on low for 3 hours, or until chicken is cooked through.
2. Remove chicken from slow-cooker and slice into strips.
3. Serve fajitas in tortillas with desired toppings.

## Nutrition:

- 354 calories
- 13g fat
- 2.3g fiber
- 41.2g protein

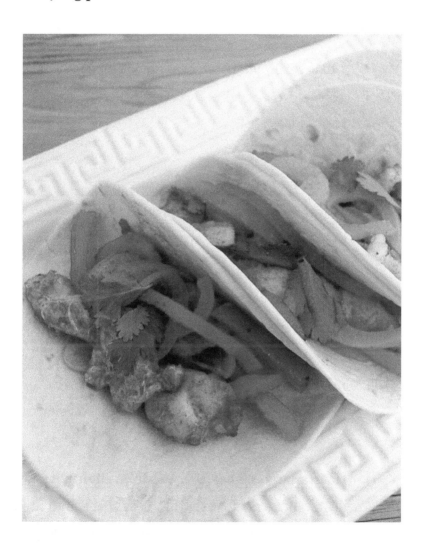

# Spring Beef Bourguignon

**Preparation Time:** 10 minutes

**Cooking Time:** 6 hours

**Servings:** 6

**Ingredients:**

- 4 lb. beef chuck roast, cut into chunks
- 3 tbsp. extra-virgin olive oil
- 1 c. red wine
- 1/2 c. beef broth
- 2 c. sliced baby bell mushrooms
- 2 large carrots, sliced into rounds
- 1 large onion, diced
- 2 cloves garlic, chopped
- 3 sprigs fresh thyme
- 3 sprigs fresh rosemary
- 1 tsp. salt - ½ tsp. pepper
- 1 bunch asparagus, trimmed and quartered
- Chopped fresh parsley, for serving

**Directions:**

1. Heat a large skillet over medium-high heat. While it heats, toss beef with oil. Sear beef in batches, 3 minutes per side. Between each batch, deglaze pan

with some red wine, scraping up any bits with a wooden spoon.

2. Pour mixture into slow-cooker along with seared beef as it's done. To slow-cooker, add beef broth, mushrooms, carrots, onion, garlic, thyme, rosemary, salt, pepper and remaining red wine.

3. Cook on high 6 hours, until beef is tender. Thirty minutes before serving, remove herbs and add asparagus; cook until just tender. Garnish with parsley and serve.

## Nutrition:

- 613 calories
- 39g fat
- 49g protein

# Mexican Shredded Beef

**Preparation Time:** 10 minutes

**Cooking Time:** 9 hours

**Servings:** 10

**Ingredients:**

- 3 pounds beef chuck roast
- 1 onion, diced
- 4 garlic cloves, minced
- 2 tablespoons tomato paste
- Juice of one lime (1-2 tablespoons)
- 1 Tablespoon chili powder
- 1 teaspoon cumin
- 1 teaspoon paprika
- 1 teaspoon dried oregano
- 1 teaspoon kosher salt, plus more to taste
- 1/4 teaspoon red chili flakes

**Directions:**

1. Mix together the chili powder, cumin, paprika, salt, oregano and red chili flakes, set aside. Add the chopped onion and garlic to the slow cooker with the tomato paste, lime juice, and just 1-2 teaspoons of the spice mixture. Stir everything together until fully mixed.

2. Sprinkle the rest of the spices all over the chuck roast, patting to help it stick to the meat.

3. Place the meat on top of the onion mixture and set cook on low for 7-8 hours. Total cooking time will vary for different roasts.

4. After meat has cooked, use two forks to shred the meat, removing any large pieces of fat or gristle as you find them. (If the meat is still too tough to shred, it needs to be cooked a little longer. Cook for an additional 30-60 minutes and check it again.) Stir to mix well with the sauce. Cover and continue to cook on low for another 30-60 minutes.

5. Before serving stir well again to mix the meat with the sauce. Taste meat and season with more salt to taste.

**Nutrition:**

- 416 calories
- 27g fat
- 28g protein

# Pork Tenderloin

**Preparation Time:** 10 minutes

**Cooking Time:** 8 hours

**Servings:** 6

**Ingredients:**

*Shredded pork:*

- 3 lbs. Pork Tenderloin
- Salt/Pepper
- Olive Oil
- 1 Cup Chicken or Vegetable Stock
- 1/2 teaspoon Ground Sage

*For blackberry sauce:*

- 10 ounces Fresh Blackberries
- 1/4 Cup Balsamic Vinegar
- 1/4 Cup Olive Oil
- Pinch Salt

**Directions:**

1. Salt and pepper pork tenderloin. Sear pork in large pan over high heat. Oil the bottom of a 6qt slow cooker.

2. Transfer pork tenderloin to slow cooker. Add stock and sage.

3. Cook on low for 8-9 hours. (I do not recommend cooking on high as it can cause the pork to dry out). Remove pork from slow cooker and shred. It should be falling apart. Pulse blackberries in blender. Push blackberry mixture through mesh strainer. Discard seeds.

4. In a 3.5qt pot, bring blackberry pulp, vinegar, olive oil and salt to a boil. Reduce heat and simmer 15-20 minutes while whisking occasionally. Vigorously whisk the last 2-3 minutes.

5. Once the sauce reaches a syrupy consistency, set aside to cool and thicken for 10 minutes before serving.

**Nutrition:**

- 188 calories
- 11g fat
- 30g protein

# Creamy Lemon Chicken

**Preparation Time:** 10 minutes

**Cooking Time:** 5 hours

**Servings:** 6

**Ingredients:**

- 5 chicken breasts boneless and skinless
- 6 tablespoons unsalted butter divided
- 1/2 teaspoon kosher salt
- 1/4 teaspoon coarse ground black pepper
- 1 teaspoon Italian seasoning
- 2 lemons juiced and zested
- 2 garlic cloves minced
- 1 cup half and half
- 1 tablespoon heavy cream.
- 1 tablespoon chicken base optional

**Directions:**

1. In a large cast iron skillet add 1 tablespoon of butter to melt on medium high heat. Add the kosher salt, black pepper and Italian seasoning to the chicken and add it to the pan.

2. Cook on each side for 4-6 minutes. Add the chicken to your slow cooker. Cover with lemon juice, lemon zest, garlic and the rest of the butter in pieces

3. Cook on low for 4 hours or on high for 2 hours. In a large measuring cup add the half and half, heavy cream and chicken base and whisk well. Add the liquid, mix, and cook an additional hour on high.

**Nutrition:**

- 465 calories
- 21g fat
- 50g protein

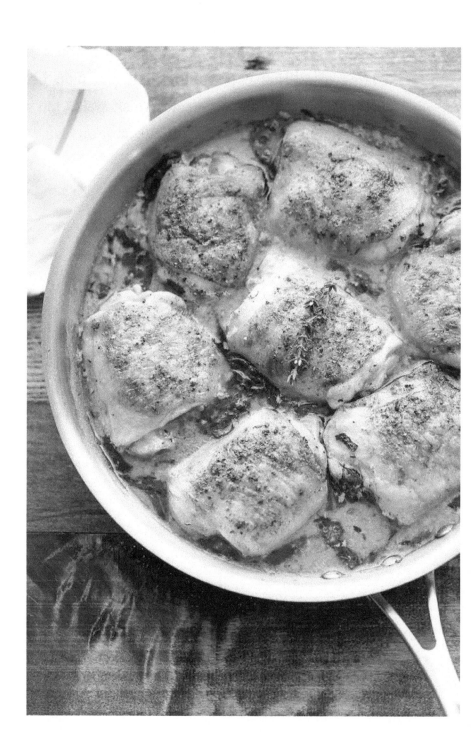

# Asian Porkchops

**Preparation Time:** 10 minutes

**Cooking Time:** 6 hours

**Servings:** 5

**Ingredients:**

- 4 thick-cut boneless pork chops
- 1 small onion, chopped
- ½ c. low-sodium soy sauce
- 2 tbsp. Splenda
- ¼ tsp. ginger

**Directions:**

1. Add pork chops and onions to the crock pot. In a small bowl, mix soy sauce, Splenda and ginger. Pour over pork chops in the crock pot. Cook on low for 6 hours or high for 3-4 hours.
2. May need to cook a little longer if your chops are frozen.

**Nutrition:**

- 306 calories
- 15g fat
- 24g protein

# Sausage and Peppers

**Preparation Time:** 10 minutes

**Cooking Time:** 6 hours

**Servings:** 6

**Ingredients:**

- 5 to 6 medium cloves garlic finely chopped
- 2 large yellow onions halved and thinly sliced
- 4 green bell peppers halved from top to bottom, cleaned and thinly sliced
- 1 tablespoon kosher salt
- 1 teaspoon Italian Seasoning
- 1/4 teaspoon dried oregano
- 1/2 teaspoon crushed red pepper flakes
- 28 ounce can unsalted crushed tomatoes
- 1/4 cup cold water
- 1 bay leaf
- 1 3/4 to 2 pounds uncooked Italian Sausage Links Mild or Spicy
- chopped Italian parsley for serving optional

**Directions:**

1. Finely chop garlic. Remove the chopped garlic and onion to the slow cooker Slice bell peppers in half from top to bottom. Remove the ribs and any seeds. Add the

sliced bell peppers to the slow cooker along with the salt, Italian Seasoning, dried oregano, crushed red pepper flakes, 1/4 cup cold water and 1 can have crushed tomatoes. Toss until well coated and liquid is evenly distributed.

2.  Remove about half of the peppers and onion mixture to a bowl. Bury the uncooked sausages in the middle and return the peppers and onions back to the slow cooker to cover the sausage. Add the bay leaf. Cover, set to low and cook for 6 hours.

3.  The onions and peppers will give off a lot of water as they cook which will make the sauce liquid and spoon-able so don't stress that there isn't enough liquid. Top with some chopped parsley, serve hot and enjoy!

**Nutrition:**

- 381 calories
- 23g fat
- 33g protein

# Low-Carb Beef Short Ribs

**Preparation Time:** 15 minutes

**Cooking Time:** 4 hours

**Servings:** 12

**Ingredients:**

- 4 lbs. boneless or bone in, beef short ribs cut crosswise into 2-inch pieces
- salt
- pepper
- 2 tbsp. olive oil
- 1 cup beef broth
- 1 cup onion chopped
- 3 cloves garlic minced
- 2 tbsp. Worcestershire sauce homemade
- 2 tbsp. tomato paste
- 1 cup red wine

**Directions:**

1. Heat the oil in a large skillet over medium high heat. Season one side of your short ribs generously with salt and pepper.
2. Place half of the ribs, seasoned side down onto the hot skillet and brown. Season the top of the ribs in the skillet with salt and pepper. Flip once the bottom is

browned. Remove and set aside while browning the rest of the meat.

3. Add beef broth to slow cooker and place short ribs into. To the same skillet add your remaining ingredients and bring to a boil. Cook for 5 minutes or until onion is tender. Pour this over the ribs in the slow-cooker. Cover and cook on high 4-6 hours or low 8-10 hours.

**Nutrition:**

- 604 calories
- 34g fat
- 5g carbs
- 65g protein

# Keto Bread

**Preparation Time:** 5 minutes

**Cooking Time:** 25 minutes

**Servings:** 6

**Ingredients:**

- 5 tablespoons butter, at room temperature, divided
- 6 large eggs, lightly beaten
- 1½ cups almond flour
- 3 teaspoons baking powder
- 1 scoop MCT oil powder
- Pinch pink Himalayan salt

**Directions:**

1. Preheat the oven to 390°F. Coat a 9-by-5-inch loaf pan with 1 tablespoon of butter. In a large bowl, use a hand mixer to mix the eggs, almond flour, remaining 4 tablespoons of butter, baking powder, MCT oil powder (if using), and pink Himalayan salt until thoroughly blended. Pour into the prepared pan.
2. Bake for 25 minutes, or until a toothpick inserted in the center comes out clean. Slice and serve.

## Nutrition:

- 165 Calories
- 15g Total Fat
- 2g Fiber
- 6g Protein

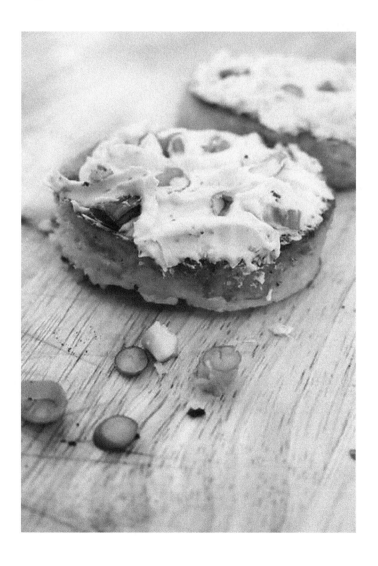

# Keto Tortilla Chips

**Preparation Time:** 5 minutes

**Cooking Time:** 5 minutes

**Servings:** 36 pieces

**Ingredients:**

*Tortilla Chips:*

- 6 flax seed tortillas
- 3 tbsp. Oil for deep frying, (absorbed oil)
- Salt and pepper to taste

*Toppings:*

- Diced jalapeno
- Fresh salsa
- Shredded cheese
- Full-fat sour cream

**Directions:**

1. Make the flaxseed tortilla's using this recipe. I get 6 total tortillas when using a tortilla press.
2. Cut the tortillas into chip-sized slices. I got 6 out of each tortilla.
3. Heat the deep fryer. Once ready, lay out the pieces of tortilla in the basket. You can fry 4-6 pieces at a time.

Fry for about 1-2 minutes, then flip. Continue to fry for another 1-2 minutes on the other side.

4. Remove from the fryer and place on paper towels to cool. Season with salt and pepper to taste. Serve with toppings of choice!

**Nutrition:**

- 40.34 Calories
- 3.03g Fats
- 0.37g Net Carbs
- 0.83g Protein.

# Flavored Keto Cheese Chips

**Preparation Time:** 10 minutes

**Cooking Time:** 5 minutes

**Servings:** 15

**Ingredients:**

- 1 ½ cups shredded cheddar cheese
- 3 tablespoons ground flaxseed meal
- Seasonings of Your Choice

**Directions:**

1. Preheat your oven to 425°F. Start by forming 2 Tbsp. Cheddar Cheese into small mounds on your non-stick pan. You want to spread them out a little bit as they will melt and expand as they're cooking.

2. In a small ramekin, measure out 3 Tbsp. Flaxseed Meal. Use this to distribute the flax evenly among all the chips you're  making. Add the seasonings of your choice to the chips! In this batch we're making 3 different flavors.

3. The first flavor is paprika and cumin. I have large spice containers for these 2, as I use them a lot. I poured them straight onto the chip and probably used more than I should have. Lesson learned: sprinkle the spices on with your fingers.

4. The second flavor is southwest chipotle and cheddar. I am using Tone's Southwest Chipotle Seasoning, one that I think is a must-have in every pantry.
5. The third, and last, flavor is a blend of onion powder, garlic powder, chili, celery seed and a few others.
6. Once all the chips are seasoned to your liking, put them in the oven for 10 minutes. They shouldn't look crisp when you take them out, but you will see little holes forming in the chips where the oil is pooling on the top.
7. Remove the chips from the oven and let them cool for 1-2 minutes. They'll start to get hard and form into the crispy chips we want. If you want to form them into different shapes, you can do that here – but be quick!
8. Transfer the chips to a paper towel to quickly get rid of excess grease. Once finished, transfer them to a platter plate. You can put salsa in the middle and serve as an appetizer or snack.

**Nutrition:**

- 65.83 Calories
- 5.27g Fats
- 3.61g Protein.

# Smoked Salmon and Goat Cheese Bites

**Preparation Time:** 10 minutes

**Cooking Time:** 15 minutes

**Servings:** 16

**Ingredients:**

- 8 ounces goat cheese, softened
- 1 tablespoon fresh oregano
- 1 tablespoon fresh rosemary
- 1 tablespoon fresh basil
- 2 cloves garlic
- Salt and pepper to taste
- 6 ounces radicchio
- 4 ounces smoked salmon

**Directions:**

1. Finely mince the oregano, rosemary, and fresh basil. Finely grate the garlic. Add the goat cheese, herbs, garlic, salt, and pepper to a mixing bowl. Combine well then set aside.

2. Cut the stem off the bottom of the radicchio. Carefully peel apart the leaves until you have 16 leaves for serving. You can save any leftover radicchio for other salads or recipes. Wash the leaves then dry them.

3. On each radicchio leave lay a piece of smoked salmon then a ½ ounce of the herbed goat cheese. Sprinkle some black pepper across the top then serve.

**Nutrition:**

- 46.19 Calories
- 3.33g Fats
- 3.43g Protein.

# Low Carb Fried Mac & Cheese

**Preparation Time:** 5 minutes

**Cooking Time:** 10 minutes

**Servings:** 5

**Ingredients:**

- 1 medium cauliflower, riced
- 1 ½ cups shredded cheddar cheese
- 3 large eggs
- 2 teaspoons paprika
- 1 teaspoon turmeric
- ¾ teaspoon rosemary

**Directions:**

1. Get your head of cauliflower ready. We'll need to prep it before ricing it. Cut your cauliflower into florets, making sure you get any excess stem off. Add the cauliflower to your food processor and pulse it until it is the consistency of short grain rice. Put your cauliflower into a microwave safe bowl, and microwave for 5-7 minutes.

2. Once it's done in the microwave, we want to get all the excess  moisture out. I lay my cauliflower onto a kitchen towel to wring it out. You will get cauliflower "juice" all over the towel, so this will need to go into

the laundry afterward. If you don't want to do that, you can do this with paper towels also.

3. Once you have the cauliflower in the kitchen towel, roll it up tight and apply pressure (your whole-body weight) to the cauliflower. Try to push as much extra moisture out of the cauliflower as you can.

4. Once you're finished, extract the "mushed" cauliflower from the kitchen towel and put it into a bowl. Make sure that its room temperature by this point.

5. Add your eggs ONE AT A TIME to the cauliflower. You don't want a mixture that too watery! Keep in mind that I only did 1/3 of the entire recipe. Add your cheese.

6. Finally, your spices to the cauliflower – turmeric, rosemary, and paprika. Mix everything well, using your hands if you want.

7. In a pan, heat your olive oil and coconut oil on high until it gets very hot. Form your cauliflower mixture into a ball, and then flatten it out in the palm of your hand. Add your cauliflower "patties" into the hot oil and reduce the heat to medium high.

8. Allow them to get crisp on one side before flipping them. Continue cooking them until they're crisp on both sides. All done! Serve on a bed of spinach, or just eat as a snack. They're absolutely delicious!

**Nutrition:**

- 39.67 Calories
- 2.71g Fats
- 2.59g Protein.

# Feta and Bacon Bites

**Preparation Time:** 10 minutes

**Cooking Time:** 15 minutes

**Servings:** 24

**Ingredients:**

- ¾ cup almond flour
- 2 cups mozzarella cheese, shredded
- 8 slices cooked bacon
- ¼ cup feta cheese, crumbled
- ¼ cup green onions, chopped
- 3 tablespoons sriracha mayo, like Sarayo
- Salt and pepper to taste

**Directions:**

1. Preheat your oven to 350°F. In a nonstick pan over medium heat, combine your almond flour and mozzarella. Stir constantly. Your flour/cheese mix will form a dough like consistency after about 5 minutes.

2. Place your dough between two pieces of parchment paper. Roll flat with a rolling pin. Use a cookie cutter or glass to cut out 24 circles.

3. If you run out of dough then form the remaining bits into a ball. Heat it up on stove, then roll it out again.

4. Place the circles of dough into your muffin tin (or on a cookie sheet.) Top with the bacon, feta, and onions. Bake at 350°F for about 15 minutes, until the edges are browned. Cool, peel off the liners, and top with sriracha mayo!

## Nutrition:

- 71.79 Calories
- 5.74g Fats
- 3.66g Protein.

# Low Carb Flax Bread

**Preparation Time:** 10 minutes

**Cooking Time:** 20 minutes

**Servings:** 8

**Ingredients:**

- 200 g ground flax seeds
- ½ cup psyllium husk powder
- 1 tablespoon baking powder
- 1 ½ cups soy protein isolate
- ¼ cup granulated Stevia
- 2 teaspoons salt
- 7 large egg whites
- 1 large whole egg
- 3 tablespoons butter
- ¾ cup water

**Directions:**

1. Preheat oven to 350°F. Mix psyllium husk, baking powder, protein isolate, sweetener, and salt together.
2. In a separate bowl, mix the egg, egg whites, butter, and water together. If you decide to add extracts or syrups, add these here! Slowly add wet ingredients to dry ingredients while mixing them.

3. Grease bread pan. Add all ingredients to the bread pan. Bake for 15-20 minutes until set.

**Nutrition:**

- 265.5 Calories
- 15.68g Fats
- 24.34g Protein.

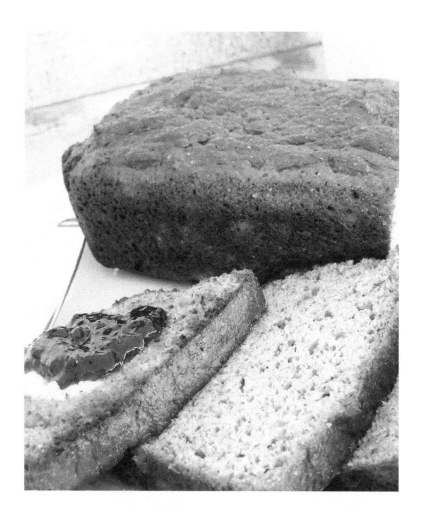

# Crispy & Delicious Kale Chips

**Preparation Time:** 5 minutes

**Cooking Time:** 15 minutes

**Servings:** 8

**Ingredients:**

- 1 large bunch kale
- 2 tablespoons olive oil
- 1 tablespoon seasoned salt

**Directions:**

1. Preheat your oven to 350°F. Remove your bindings on your bunch of kale. Separate the leaves from the stems of your kale. You want to try to get as little stem as possible. Rinse your kale with cold water. Add it to your vegetable spinner and remove as much water as possible.

2. Add your kale to a kitchen towel and remove excess water drops. Put your kale into a Ziploc bag and add 1 Tbsp. Olive Oil. Mix it well so that it coats every single leaf.

3. Add your kale to a baking sheet. You want to make sure that the kale is spread out a little bit. Try to press the leaves flat so you get a more even and crisped cook on each leaf.

4. Bake the kale for 12 minutes and remove from the oven. You want the edges of the kale to be a little browned, but the rest of the kale to stay a darkish green.

5. BE CAREFUL – there is a fine line between being overcooked and being perfect. When they're overcooked, they come out very bitter.

6. Add your salt to the finished kale and serve! You can add different seasonings, or just use your favorite seasoned salt.

## Nutrition:

- 80.5 Calories
- 7.15g Fats
- 1.82g Protein.

# Low Carb Broccoli and Cheese Fritters

**Preparation Time:** 10 minutes

**Cooking Time:** 5 minutes

**Servings:** 16

**Ingredients:**

*The Fritters:*

- ¾ cup almond flour
- 7 tablespoons flaxseed meal
- 4 ounces fresh broccoli
- 4 ounces mozzarella cheese
- 2 large eggs
- 2 teaspoons baking powder
- Salt and Pepper to taste

*The Sauce:*

- ¼ cup mayonnaise
- ¼ cup fresh chopped dill
- ½ tablespoon lemon juice
- Salt and pepper to taste

**Directions:**

1. Add broccoli to a food processor and pulse until the broccoli is broken down into small pieces. You want it to be well processed. Mix together the cheese, almond

flour, ¼ cup flaxseed meal and baking powder with the broccoli.

2. If you want to add any extra seasonings (salt and pepper), do it at this point.

3. Add the 2 eggs and mix together well until everything is incorporated. Roll the batter into balls and then coat with 3 tablespoons flaxseed meal. Continue doing this with all of the batter and set aside on paper towels.

4. Heat your deep fat fryer to 375F. I use this deep fat fryer. Once ready, lay broccoli and cheese fritters inside the basket, not overcrowding it.

5. Fry the fritters until golden brown, about 3-5 minutes. Once done, lay on paper towels to drain excess grease and season to your tastes. Feel free to make a zesty dill and lemon mayonnaise for a dip. Enjoy!

**Nutrition:**

- 78 Calories
- 5.8g Fats
- 4.6g Protein

# Chocolate Cobbler

**Preparation Time:** 10 minutes

**Cooking Time:** 40 minutes

**Servings:** 8

**Ingredients:**

**Chocolate Layer Ingredients:**

- 1/3 cup granulated Erythritol-based Sweetener
- 1¼ cups blanched Almond flour
- ¼ cup Cocoa powder
- 3 tbsp. of unflavored Whey Protein powder
- 2 tsp. of baking powder
- ½ tsp. of Espresso powder
- ¼ tsp. of salt
- ½ stick (¼ cup) of unsalted melted Butter
- ½ cup of heavy Whipping Cream

**Topping Ingredients:**

- 1 tbsp. of Cocoa powder
- ¾ cup of hot Water
- 2 tbsp. of granulated Erythritol-based Sweetener

**Directions:**

1. Heat the oven to 325° F. Preparing the chocolate layer: Whisk the baking powder, salt, espresso powder, protein powder, cocoa powder, sweetener, and almond flour in a large bowl until it is well mixed. In an 8-inch baking dish, evenly spread the mixture.

2. Preparing the topping: Whisk the cocoa powder and the sweetener together in a small bowl. Evenly sprinkle on the top of the cobbler. Empty the hot water over the cobbler and make sure not to stir.

3. Place in an oven and bake for 35-40 minutes until the center is set.

4. Take out of the oven and allow to cool for 10-15 minutes. Serve warm.

**Nutrition:**

- 20g Fats
- 7.1g Carbohydrates
- 6.5g Protein
- 223 Calories

# Easy Shortbread Crust

**Preparation Time:** 5 minutes

**Cooking Time:** 15 minutes

**Servings:** 10

**Ingredients:**

- ¼ cup of powdered Erythritol-based Sweetener
- 150g (1½ cups) of blanched Almond flour
- ¼ cup (½ stick) of unsalted melted Butter
- ½ tsp. of salt

**Directions:**

1. Whisk together the salt, sweetener, and almond flour in a medium dish.
2. Add the melted butter and stir until mixture starts to clump together.

**Nutrition:**

- 12.7g fats
- 3.6g Carbohydrates
- 3.7g Protein
- 137 Calories

# Keto Chocolate Kisses

**Preparation Time:** 10 minutes

**Cooking Time:** 15 minutes

**Servings:** 20

**Ingredients:**

- 2 ounces unsweetened baking chocolate
- 1 ½ tablespoons Swerve confectioners' powdered sweetener
- ¼ teaspoon vanilla extract
- A pinch stevia concentrated powder
- ½ ounce food grade cocoa butter

**Directions:**

1. Add chocolate, sweetener and cocoa butter into a heatproof bowl. Place the bowl in a double boiler. Stir occasionally until the mixture melts. You can also melt it in a small pan over low heat.
2. Add stevia and vanilla and mix well. Spoon into 20 chocolate molds. Cool completely.
3. Chill until firm. Remove from mold and serve. Leftovers can be stored in an airtight container in the refrigerator.

## Nutrition:

- 24.8 Calories
- 0.8g Carbohydrates
- 0.4g Protein

Lightning Source UK Ltd.
Milton Keynes UK
UKHW021013240621
386072UK00001B/94

9 781803 177120